10 CRUCIAL CONSIDERATIONS

TO NAVIGATING THE CARE OF YOUR AGING PARENT

EXPERT GUIDANCE, PRACTICAL ADVICE, & ESSENTIAL RESOURCES
TO PREPARE YOU FOR THE CHALLENGES OF CAREGIVING

BY
RICHELE WILKINS, RN, BSN
CEO, FOUNDER CARING HANDS HOME HEALTH, INC.

CARING HANDS HOME HEALTH, © 2024

A CARING HANDS RELIABLE RESOURCE
COPYRIGHT 2024, CARING HANDS HOME HEALTH
WWW.CARINGHANDSHHC.COM

ISBN 13: 979-8-9916-094-0-1

NOTICE OF RIGHTS

All rights reserved. No part of this book may be reproduced or transmitted in any form by any means, electronic, mechanical, photocopying, recording, or otherwise, eithout the prior written permission of the publisher or author. For information on getting permission for reprints and excerpts, contact clients@caringhandshhc.org.

NOTICE OF LIABILITY

The information in this book is distributed on an "As is" basis without warranty. While every precaution has been taken in the preparation of this book, neither the author nor publisher shall have any liability to any person or entity with respect to any loss or damage caused or alleged to be caused directly or indirectly by the instructions contained in this book.

Table of
CONTENTS

Preface IX

Chapter 1: Understanding the Mindset for Care 1

Introduction to the Mindset
Definition and importance of having the right mindset for caregiving.

Assessing Readiness
Self-assessment tools for children and parents to evaluate their preparedness for the caregiving journey.

Building Empathy
Techniques to foster empathy and understanding.

Chapter 2: Communication is Key 14

Open Dialogue
Strategies for initiating and maintaining open, honest conversations about care needs and preferences.

Active Listening
Tips for improving listening skills to better understand and respond to parents' concerns.

Conflict Resolution
Methods for resolving disagreements and finding common ground.

Chapter 3: Navigating Emotional Challenges 17

Managing Stress and Guilt
Practical advice for coping with the emotional strain of caregiving.

Support Systems
Identifying and utilizing support networks, including family, friends, and professional counselors.

Self-Care for Caregivers
Importance of self-care and strategies to maintain mental and emotional health.

Chapter 4: Understanding Medical & Health Needs — 22

Basic Medical Knowledge
Overview of common health issues in aging parents and essential medical knowledge for caregivers.

Medication Management
Best practices for managing and organizing medications.

Monitoring Health
Techniques for tracking health changes and knowing when to seek medical advice.

Chapter 5: Financial Planning and Management — 28

Budgeting for Care
Creating a budget that includes caregiving expenses.

Insurance and Benefits
Understanding and navigating healthcare insurance, Medicare, and other benefits.

Financial Assistance
Exploring options for financial aid and support programs.

Chapter 6: Balancing Work, Life, and Caregiving   35

Time Management Techniques
Strategies for efficiently managing time between work, personal life, and caregiving duties.

Employer Support
Understanding workplace policies and seeking support from employers.

Delegating Responsibilities
How to share caregiving duties with other family members or hire professional help.

Chapter 7: Legal Considerations and Planning   40

Legal Documents
Importance of wills, power of attorney, and advanced directives.

Guardianship and Conservatorship
Understanding legal options and procedures for managing an aging parent's affairs.

Estate Planning
Basics of estate planning and ensuring parents' wishes are honored.

Chapter 8: Enhancing Quality of Life   44

Activities and Engagement
Ideas for keeping aging parents mentally and physically active.

Home Modifications
Making the home safer and more comfortable for aging parents.

Social Connections
Encouraging social interaction to prevent isolation and loneliness.

Chapter 9: Keeping in Touch and Staying Happy — 54

Community Services
Overview of local community services and how to access them.

Professional Caregivers
When and how to hire professional caregiving services.

Support Groups
Finding and joining support groups for caregivers and aging parents.

Chapter 10: Planning for the Future — 58

Long-Term Care Options
Exploring different long-term care options, including assisted living and nursing homes.

End-of-Life Planning
Approaching conversations about end-of-life wishes with sensitivity and care.

Continuous Learning and Adaptation
Emphasizing the importance of ongoing learning and adapting to changing needs and circumstances.

Final Thoughts — 63

About Caring Hands Home Health — 63

About the Author — 64

PREFACE

Caregiving is an inevitable part of life for many of us, whether it's for a parent, spouse, sibling, aunt, disabled child, or even a close friend. Throughout this book, you will find the term "parent" used frequently. However, please understand that it is intended as a placeholder for anyone you may find yourself caring for in the future. The principles and insights shared here apply to a wide range of caregiving situations.

This book is designed to provide you with the basic information needed to start thinking about the responsibilities and challenges of caregiving. It's not a question of if caregiving will enter your life, but when. Being prepared can make a world of difference for both you and those you care for.

Our goal is that, by the end of this book, you will feel more informed, encouraged, and equipped to face the challenges of caregiving with dignity and grace. The journey ahead may have its hurdles, but with the right knowledge and preparation, you can navigate it successfully.

Once you've absorbed these basics, we strongly encourage you to consult with an experienced senior advisor to gain a more detailed understanding of your unique situation. The better prepared you are, the better off everyone involved will be.

- Richele Wilkins
  CEO, Founder of Caring Hands Home Health, Inc.

CHAPTER 1

UNDERSTANDING THE MINDSET FOR CARE

Taking care of older parents is a big and often difficult job. It requires more than just knowing what to do—it's just as important to be kind and resilient. Having a caring and tough attitude may be the most important part of doing a good job as a caregiver. And it can help both you and your parents feel better about a caregiver situation, making the whole experience better for everyone.

The right attitude for taking care of parents includes being kind, patient, and ready to help. It means understanding how your parents feel and what they need. You should be ready to meet their needs with attention and respect. Having the right attitude helps you do your job with purpose and commitment, making the care you give infinitely better.

Before you start taking care of your parents, it's important to see if you're ready. This means thinking about how you feel and if you can handle the job. There are tools that can help you figure this out. These tools provide statements that help you determine what you're good at and where you might need to improve. For example, you will be asked to consider how stressed you are, how much time you have, and how well you can handle problems.

It's also important to talk to your parents about this. You need to know if they are ready to accept help and what kind of help they need. Working together like this ensures everyone is on the same page and can work well together.

ASSESSING YOUR READINESS FOR CAREGIVING

Below and on the following pages, you will find the Caregiver Preparedness and Mindset Assessment. Please take this assessment with an open mind and with as much honesty as possible. The assessment will focus on the caregiving role for aging parents, but the word "parent" can be exchanged to encompass any caregiving situation.

Assess your readiness for caregiving by indicating whether you agree or disagree with each statement.

AGREE / DISAGREE

EMOTIONAL & MENTAL PREPAREDNESS

1. I am comfortable with the idea of taking on a caregiver role for my parents.
2. I am sure I can handle seeing my parents' health decline without becoming overwhelmed.
3. I can provide emotional support and comfort to my parents.
4. I can handle the emotional toll of caregiving without it negatively affecting my relationship with my parents.
5. I can remain patient and calm in stressful situations.
6. I am ready and willing to adapt to the changing circumstances of my parents' evolving needs.
7. I find it easy to empathize with my parents' experiences and emotions.
8. I am ready to provide care with compassion and understanding, even when it's challenging.
9. I am committed to taking care of my own physical and mental health while caregiving.
10. I have strategies in place to manage stress and prevent burnout.

AGREE DISAGREE

COMMUNICATION & RELATIONSHIPS

☐ ☐ 11. I am comfortable discussing sensitive topics like health, finances, and end-of-life care with my parents.

☐ ☐ 12. I can effectively communicate with healthcare professionals and advocate for my parents' needs.

☐ ☐ 13. I can resolve conflicts with my parents or other family members constructively.

☐ ☐ 14. I can navigate disagreements about care decisions calmly and effectively.

☐ ☐ 15. I am willing to respect my parent's desire to maintain their independence as much as possible.

☐ ☐ 16. I am willing to involve my parents in decisions about their care.

☐ ☐ 17. I can adjust my caregiving approach based on feedback from my parents and healthcare providers.

☐ ☐ 18. I am open to trying new methods and strategies to improve care.

☐ ☐ 19. I have a support system of family, friends, or professional caregivers to help me.

☐ ☐ 20. I am open to seeking support from caregiver support groups or counseling if needed.

SKILLS & KNOWLEDGE

☐ ☐ 21. I have basic knowledge of common health issues that affect older adults.

☐ ☐ 22. I can learn new skills, such as medication management and mobility assistance, to care for my parents.

☐ ☐ 23. I understand my parents' medical conditions and treatments.

☐ ☐ 24. I can recognize signs of health problems and know when to seek medical help.

☐ ☐ 25. I can effectively troubleshoot and resolve problems that arise during caregiving.

☐ ☐ 26. I am resourceful in finding solutions and support when needed.

☐ ☐ 27. I am organized and able to keep track of medical appointments, medications, and caregiving tasks.

☐ ☐ 28. I have a system in place for managing important documents and information.

AGREE	DISAGREE	
☐	☐	29. I am fully committed to the responsibilities of caregiving, even when it becomes difficult.
☐	☐	30. I understand that caregiving might be a long-term commitment.

PLANNING & LOGISTICS

AGREE	DISAGREE	
☐	☐	31. I have enough time in my schedule to dedicate to caregiving duties.
☐	☐	32. I am willing to adjust my current lifestyle to accommodate caregiving responsibilities.
☐	☐	33. My home, and/or my parents' home, is safe and accessible for their current and future needs.
☐	☐	34. I am willing to make necessary modifications to ensure their comfort and safety.
☐	☐	35. I have considered how I will manage if my parents' care needs increase over time.
☐	☐	36. I am prepared to seek additional help or transition to professional care if necessary.
☐	☐	37. I have considered the financial impact of caregiving, including potential medical expenses.
☐	☐	38. I am aware of financial resources and assistance programs available for caregivers.
☐	☐	39. I have discussed and documented my parents' preferences for long-term care and end-of-life decisions.
☐	☐	40. I am prepared to adjust plans as my parent's needs change over time.

After you've completed this 40 question assessment, count the number of questions to which you responded "DISAGREE" and place that number in the box below.

☐ **TOTAL DISAGREE**

UNDERSTANDING YOUR ASSESSMENT RESULTS

This assessment is a litmus test of your readiness to be a caregiver for your aging parent or loved one. It addresses 20 key areas that are crucial to your success as a caregiver.

If you disagreed with between 1 and 5 statements, you are moderately prepared for your role as a caregiver to your aging parent. There are areas, however, that you will need to learn, grow, or prepare for to be most successful in your role.

If you disagreed with between 6-10 statements, you are slightly prepared to care for your aging loved one. You have a decent number of the bases covered, but there are some important gaps that must be filled to succeed as a caregiver.

If you disagreed with 11 or more of the statements, you are unprepared to care for you aging loved one at this time. The higher that number is, the more unprepared you are at this time. There are significant gaps, skills, adjustments and preparation that need to take place in order to successfully care for your loved one in a caregiver role.

Note that all statements reflect crucial components of the caregiver existence and role. Even one statement with an answer of "DISAGREE" indicates an area that you need to grow in, learn, or prepare for in order to be successful as a caregiver and ensure your parents' happiness and well-being.

DIGGING DEEPER

The following reflects the key areas each of the statements correspond with. The good news is that this book touches on each of these key areas. If you disagreed with any of the statements, be sure to read the section of this book that discusses that key area in order to gain better understanding and insights into how to close those gaps.

- Statements 1 & 2 .... Emotional Readiness .... Chapter 1
- Statements 3 & 4 .... Emotional Support .... Chapter 3
- Statements 5 & 6 .... Patience & Flexibility .... Chapter 2
- Statements 7 & 8 .... Empathy and Compassion .... Chapter 1
- Statements 9 & 10 ..... Self-care Chapter3
- Statements 11 & 12 ..... Communication .... Chapter 2
- Statements 13 & 14 .... Conflict Resolution .... Chapter 2
- Statements 15 & 16 .... Respect for Autonomy .... Chapter 1
- Statements 17 & 18 .... Adaptability .... Chapter 6
- Statements 19 & 20 ... Support System .... Chapter 3
- Statements 21 & 22 ... Knowledge & Skills .... Chapter 4
- Statements 23 & 24 ... Medical Knowledge .... Chapter 4
- Statements 25 & 26 ... Problem-Solving .... Chapter 2
- Statements 27 & 28 ... Organization .... Chapter 7
- Statements 29 & 30 ... Commitment .... Chapter 1
- Statements 31 & 32 .....Time Management .... Chapter 6
- Statements 33 & 34 ....Home Environment .... Chapter 8
- Statements 35 & 36 ....Future Care Needs .... Chapter 10
- Statements 37 & 38 ....Financial Preparedness .... Chapter 5
- Statements 39 & 40 ....Long-Term Planning .... Chapter 10

EMPATHY IS IMPORTANT

Empathy means understanding how other people feel. It's very important for caregivers. When caregivers put themselves in their parents' shoes, they can better understand what their parents are going through.

6

You can build empathy by listening carefully and talking openly with your parents. When you actively listen to their worries and fears, you can take better care of them. Here are some ways to demonstrate empathy.

- **Active Listening**: Spend time listening to your parents' concerns, fears, and memories without interruption. This shows that you value their feelings and experiences.

- **Patience**: Understand that tasks may take longer for your parents and be patient with them. Avoid rushing or showing frustration.

- **Respecting Their Wishes**: Respect your parents' choices and preferences, even if they differ from your own. This includes decisions about their care and daily activities.

- **Regular Check-Ins**: Frequently check in with your parents to see how they're feeling and if they need anything. This shows you care about their well-being.

- **Helping with Tasks**: Assist with daily tasks such as cooking, cleaning, or shopping, especially those that have become difficult for them. This can ease their burden and show your support.

- **Encouraging Independence**: Allow your parents to do as much as they can on their own to maintain their sense of independence and dignity.

- **Sharing Activities**: Engage in activities that your parents enjoy, like playing games, watching movies, or going for walks. This shows that you value spending quality time with them.

- **Learning About Their Health**: Educate yourself about any medical conditions your parents have. Understanding their health issues can help you better support and empathize with their experiences.

- **Emotional Support**: Be there for your parents emotionally, offering comfort and reassurance during difficult times. Acknowledge their feelings and provide a shoulder to lean on.

These actions demonstrate empathy by considering your parents' emotions, respecting their autonomy, and showing them consistent care and understanding.

Learning about aging and common health problems older people face can also make you more empathetic. Knowing what happens as people get older can help you know what your parents need and how to help them.

As people age, their bodies go through various changes that can lead to common health problems. Aging often brings about decreased bone density, leading to conditions like osteoporosis, which increases the risk of fractures. Arthritis is another common issue, causing joint pain and stiffness. Heart disease and high blood pressure become more prevalent, as well as diabetes. Cognitive decline, including memory loss and dementia, can affect mental sharpness. Vision and hearing impairments are also common. Regular health check-ups, a balanced diet, exercise, and preventive measures can help manage and mitigate these health problems, improving quality of life for older adults.

KEEPING A POSITIVE ATTITUDE

Having a positive attitude is very important when taking care of your parents. It helps you handle challenges with hope and strength. Caregiving can be hard, but staying positive can stop you from feeling too stressed and help you have a better relationship with your parents.

Focus on the good things about being a caregiver. Taking care of your parents can make your family closer and create special memories. Celebrating small wins and noticing the "good" things can make you feel better and keep you motivated.

BEING PROACTIVE AND FLEXIBLE

Being proactive means planning ahead. This helps you avoid problems and be ready for unexpected turns. You can do this by keeping up with your parents' health, going to doctor's appointments, and making your home safe.

Being flexible is also very important. You need to be ready to change plans if your parents' needs change. This might mean asking for help from other caregivers or using community services. Here are some community resources that can help when caring for elderly parents:

- **Area Agencies on Aging (AAA)**: Local organizations that provide services such as meal delivery, transportation, and caregiver support.

- **Adult Day Care Centers**: Facilities that offer social activities, meals, and health services for seniors during the day, providing respite for caregivers.

- **Senior Centers**: Community centers that offer social, recreational, and educational activities for seniors.

- **Meals on Wheels**: A program that delivers nutritious meals to homebound seniors.

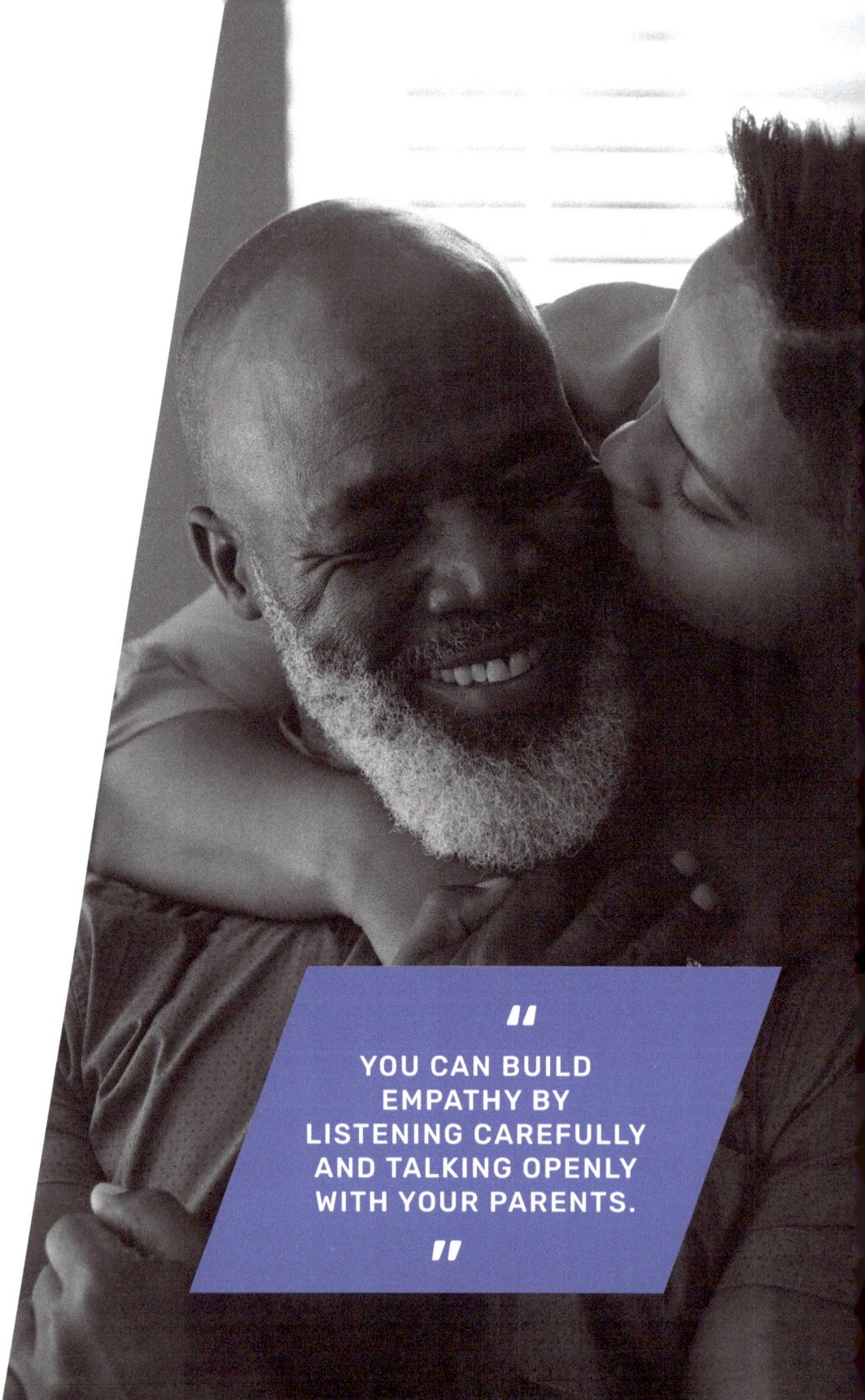

- **Home Health Care Services**: Agencies that provide medical and non-medical in-home care, including nursing, physical therapy, and personal care assistance.

- **Respite Care Programs**: Services that provide temporary relief for primary caregivers by offering short-term care for elderly parents.

- **Transportation Services**: Local transportation services for seniors, often provided by community organizations, can help with getting to medical appointments, shopping, and social activities.

- **Support Groups**: Groups that offer emotional support and practical advice for caregivers. These can be found through hospitals, community centers, or online.

- **Hospice and Palliative Care Services**: Organizations that provide end-of-life care and support for both patients and their families.

- **Legal Aid Services**: Organizations that offer free or low-cost legal assistance for seniors on issues such as wills, power of attorney, and elder rights.

- **Local Health Departments**: Organizations that often provide information on available health services, immunizations, and wellness programs for seniors.

- **Nonprofit Organizations**: Many nonprofits, such as the Alzheimer's Association or the Arthritis Foundation, offer resources, support, and information specific to certain conditions.

- **Faith-Based Organizations**: Churches, synagogues, and other faith-based organizations often offer support services, including visitation programs and caregiver support groups.

- **Public Libraries**: Libraries may offer resources on caregiving, including books, DVDs, and sometimes workshops or seminars.

- **Veterans Affairs (VA)**: If your parent is a veteran, the VA offers various health care services, financial assistance, and caregiver support programs.

- **Geriatric Care Managers**: Professionals who can help manage, coordinate, and advocate for the care of elderly parents, often offering personalized care plans.

- **Social Services**: Local social services departments may provide assistance with finding and applying for benefits, such as Medicaid or Supplemental Security Income (SSI).

- **Community Health Clinics**: Clinics that provide medical, dental, and mental health services on a sliding scale based on income.

- **Volunteer Programs**: Programs that connect volunteers with seniors for companionship, home repairs, or errands.

- **Educational Workshops**: Many community organizations offer workshops on topics such as dementia care, financial planning, and health care navigation.

These resources can provide valuable support, helping to ease the burden of caregiving and ensuring that elderly parents receive the care and attention they need.

CONCLUSION

To be a good caregiver, you need to be kind, positive, ready to help, and flexible. By checking if you're ready, building empathy, keeping a good attitude, and being proactive and flexible, you can make sure your parents get the best care. This will help both you and your parents have a better experience and stronger relationship.

CHAPTER 2

COMMUNICATION IS KEY

Communicating well is very important when taking care of your aging parents. It helps make sure everyone understands each other and works together nicely. In this chapter, we will learn how to start and keep good conversations, listen better, and solve problems.

OPEN DIALOGUE

Talking openly with your parents about their care needs can be hard, but it's very important. Start by picking a good time and place where everyone feels comfortable and can talk without distractions.

When you start the conversation, be kind and respectful. Ask questions that let your parents share their thoughts. For example, instead of asking, "Do you need help with your medications?" try asking, "How do you feel about managing your medications?" This way, they can tell you what they really think.

ACTIVE LISTENING

Listening well is a key skill for caregivers. It means paying full attention to what your parents say, understanding them, and remembering their words. Here are some tips for listening well:

- **Show Empathy**: Let your parents know you understand their feelings. You can say things like, "I understand this must be difficult for you."

- **Avoid Interrupting**: Let your parents talk without interrupting. This shows respect.

- **Clarify and Summarize**: Repeat back what your parents said in your own words to make sure you understand. For example, "So you're saying that you feel overwhelmed by managing your appointments?"

CONFLICT RESOLUTION

Disagreements can happen, but they can be solved effectively. Try to find solutions that work for both you and your parents.

Start by calmly saying how you feel using "I" statements. For example, "I feel worried when you don't take your medications on time because I want you to stay healthy." Then, listen to your parents' side of things and discuss possible solutions together.

NON-VERBAL COMMUNICATION

Body language, facial expressions, and tone of voice are also important. They can show either support and care or frustration and impatience.

Make eye contact to show you are paying attention. Use gentle movements and keep your voice calm. A warm smile or a comforting touch can also show that you care.

TECHNOLOGY AND COMMUNICATION

Today, technology can help caregivers and parents stay connected. Video calls, messaging apps, and digital calendars can be very useful. For example, a shared digital calendar can help everyone keep track of medical appointments and other important dates.

CONCLUSION

Good communication is key to successful caregiving. By talking openly, listening well, solving problems nicely, watching non-verbal cues, and using technology, caregivers can create a supportive and understanding environment. This makes sure the needs of aging parents are met and makes the caregiving journey better for everyone.

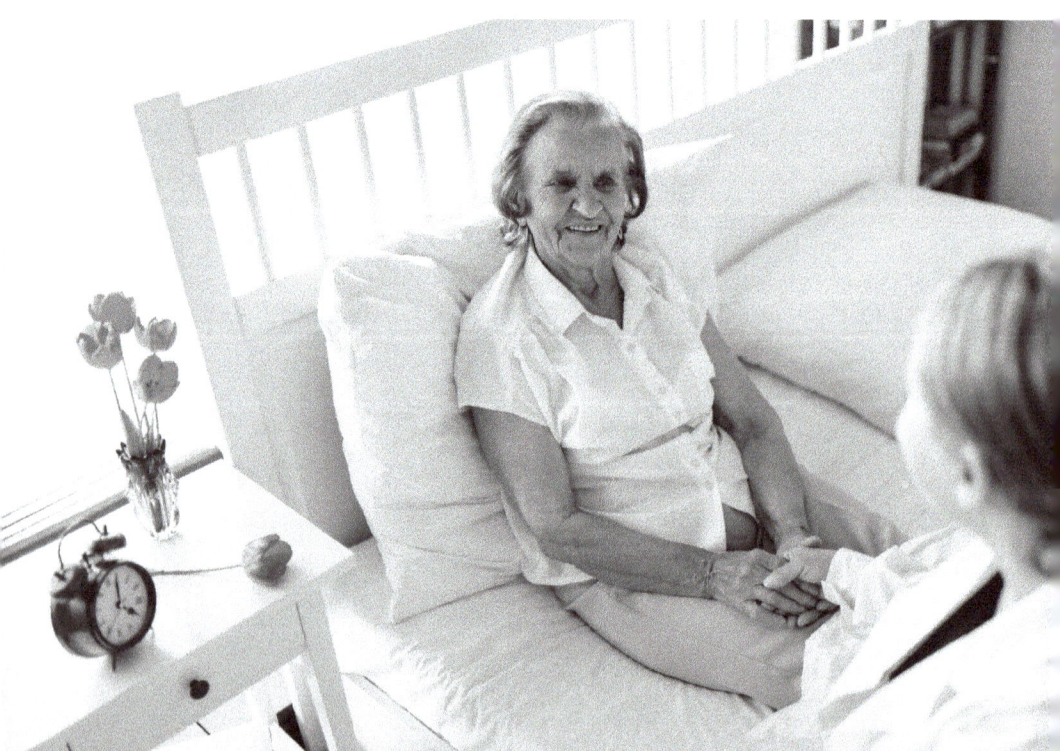

CHAPTER 3

NAVIGATING EMOTIONAL CHALLENGES

Taking care of aging parents is a big job that can cause a range of emotions. You might feel happy and affectionate, while at the same time also stressed and guilty. It's important to reconcile these feelings to keep both you and your parents happy and healthy. In this chapter, we'll learn how to manage stress and guilt, build support systems, and take care of ourselves.

MANAGING STRESS AND GUILT

Being a caregiver can sometimes feel like too much, leading to stress. You might also feel guilty, worrying that you're not doing enough. It's important to recognize these feelings and deal with them so you don't burn out.

One way to manage stress is to plan your time well. Make a schedule that balances taking care of your parents with time for yourself. Set realistic goals and learn to say "no" when you have too much to do. Remember, it's okay to ask for help.

Feeling guilty is normal, and it doesn't mean you're doing something wrong. Talk about your feelings with a friend, family member, or counselor to get some relief. Remember, no one is perfect, and doing your best really is enough.

SUPPORT SYSTEMS

You don't have to do everything alone. Having a support system can make caregiving easier. Support can come from family, friends, and professionals.

Family members can help with caregiving tasks, so the work doesn't fall on one person. Talk with your family about how they can help, whether it's through regular check-ins, financial support, or specific tasks.

Friends can offer emotional support and practical help, like running errands or giving you a break. Just having someone to talk to can make a big difference.

Professional support, like home health aides, respite care providers, and counselors, can also be very helpful. These professionals are trained to provide specific types of care and can offer support that family and friends might not be able to provide.

SELF-CARE FOR CAREGIVERS

Taking care of yourself is not just a nice thing to do—it's necessary. Self-care helps you stay healthy so you can take better care of your parents. If you ignore self-care, you might burn out, which is bad for both you and your parents.

Self-care includes physical activities like exercise and healthy eating, and mental activities like hobbies and socializing. Regular exercise, like a daily walk, can reduce stress and improve your mood. Eating nutritious meals can give you more energy.

Mental and emotional self-care means taking time to relax and do things you enjoy, like reading, gardening, painting, or spending time with friends. Mindfulness practices, like meditation and deep-breathing exercises, can also help manage stress.

NAVIGATING EMOTIONAL CHALLENGES: A CHECKLIST

Use the following checklist to help you navigate the emotional challenges that often come with caregiving.

MANAGING STRESS & GUILT

- **Recognize Your Feelings**:
  - ☐ Identify Feelings of stress and guilt.
  - ☐ Accept that these feelings are normal.
- **Create a Schedule**:
  - ☐ Balance caregiving tasks with personal time.
  - ☐ Prioritize tasks and set realistic goals.
- **Set Boundaries**:
  - ☐ Learn to say "no" to additional responsibilities when needed.
  - ☐ Delegate tasks when possible.
- **Talk About Your Feelings**:
  - ☐ Share your feelings with a trusted friend, family member, or counselor.
  - ☐ Understand that feeling guilty doesn't mean you're doing something wrong.

BUILDING SUPPORT SYSTEMS

- **Involve Family Members**:
  - ☐ Have open conversations about how they can help.
  - ☐ Divide caregiving tasks among family members.

- **Seek Help From Friends:**
  - ☐ Ask friends for emotional support and practical help.
  - ☐ Accept offers for help with errands or respite care.
- **Use Professional Services:**
  - ☐ Consider hiring home health aides or respite care providers.
  - ☐ Consult with counselors or therapists for emotional support.
- **Join Support Groups:**
  - ☐ Look for caregiver support groups in your community or online.
  - ☐ Share experiences and advice with other caregivers.

SELF-CARE FOR CAREGIVERS

- **Take Care of Your Physical Health:**
  - ☐ Engage in regular exercise, like walking or yoga.
  - ☐ Eat nutritious meals and stay hydrated.
- **Make Time for Relaxation:**
  - ☐ Schedule time for activities you enjoy, like reading or gardening.
  - ☐ Practice mindfulness, meditation, or deep-breathing exercises.
- **Maintain Social Connections:**
  - ☐ Spend time with friends and family outside of caregiving.
  - ☐ Join clubs or groups that interest you.
- **Get Enough Rest:**
  - ☐ Ensure you are getting enough sleep each night.
  - ☐ Take short breaks throughout the day to recharge.
- **Seek Professional Help if Needed:**
  - ☐ Consult a doctor or therapist if you're feeling overwhelmed.
  - ☐ Consider respite care to give yourself a break.

GENERAL TIPS

- **Stay Organized**:
  - ☐ Keep a caregiving journal or planner to track tasks and appointments.
  - ☐ Use reminders or apps to help manage your schedule.
- **Celebrate Small Wins**:
  - ☐ Acknowledge and celebrate small achievements in caregiving.
  - ☐ Reflect on positive moments to boost your morale.
- **Educate Yourself**:
  - ☐ Learn about your parents' health conditions and care needs.
  - ☐ Stay informed about caregiving resources and support available.

This checklist can help you manage the emotional challenges of caregiving, ensuring that both you and your parents stay healthy and happy.

CONCLUSION

Handling the emotional challenges of caregiving is very important for keeping both you and your parents healthy. By managing stress and guilt, building support systems, and taking care of yourself, you can make caregiving a more positive and rewarding experience. This will not only improve the care you give, but also strengthen your relationship with your parents.

CHAPTER 4

UNDERSTANDING MEDICAL AND HEALTH NEEDS

Taking care of aging parents requires your intimate understanding of their medical and health needs. This chapter will cover common health problems, managing medicines, and watching for changes in health.

BASIC MEDICAL KNOWLEDGE

As parents get older, they may have health issues that need attention. Common problems include arthritis, diabetes, heart disease, and memory issues like dementia and Alzheimer's disease. Knowing about these problems can improve your care for them.

- **Arthritis**: Arthritis causes joint pain and stiffness, making it hard to move. Helping with exercises and understanding parents' medications can be helpful for caregivers.

- **Diabetes**: Caregivers need to know how to check blood sugar levels, give insulin, and watch for signs of high or low blood sugar.

- **Heart Disease**: Parents with this may require your checking of their blood pressure, encouraging healthy eating, and recognizing signs of heart trouble.

- **Memory Issues**: Caregivers should know the stages of diseases like dementia and find ways to manage changes in behavior and communication.

Of these medical conditions, signs of dementia may be the most complex and challenging to manage. Here are real-world examples illustrating the stages of dementia:

EARLY STAGE DEMENTIA

FORGETTING APPOINTMENTS

Behavior: Jane, a 68-year-old retiree, starts forgetting her weekly book club meetings. Previously, she was always punctual and organized.

Impact: Jane feels frustrated and embarrassed when she realizes she's missed several meetings. Her friends notice but think it's just normal aging.

MISPLACING ITEMS

Behavior: John, a 72-year-old former teacher, begins misplacing everyday items like his keys and glasses more frequently. He often finds them in unusual places, like the refrigerator.

Impact: John becomes anxious and spends a lot of time looking for his lost items, which makes him late for appointments.

MIDDLE STAGE DEMENTIA

GETTING LOST IN FAMILIAR PLACES

Behavior: Mary, a 75-year-old grandmother, gets lost while walking to a nearby park she has visited daily for years.

Impact: Her family becomes worried and decides she should no longer go out alone. Mary feels a loss of independence.

TROUBLE WITH DAILY TASKS

Behavior: Bob, a 77-year-old retired engineer, struggles to follow a recipe he has cooked many times. He forgets ingredients and steps, resulting in incomplete meals.

Impact: Bob's wife starts supervising his cooking, but he feels upset and confused about why he can't remember something so familiar.

LATE STAGE DEMENTIA

DIFFICULTY COMMUNICATING

Behavior: Sarah, an 80-year-old former artist, has trouble finding the right words and often speaks in fragmented sentences. She becomes easily frustrated during conversations.

Impact: Her family has to guess what she means and help her express herself, which leads to shorter and less frequent interactions.

DEPENDENCE ON CARE

Behavior: Tom, an 82-year-old who loved gardening, now needs help with almost all daily activities, including bathing, dressing, and eating.

Impact: His daughter becomes his full-time caregiver, helping with every aspect of his life. Tom often seems confused and sometimes doesn't recognize his family members.

END STAGE DEMENTIA

SEVERE COGNITIVE DECLINE

Behavior: Alice, an 85-year-old, is mostly bedridden and unresponsive. She can no longer speak, walk, or recognize her family.

Impact: Alice requires round-the-clock care in a nursing home. Her family visits regularly, but Alice is unable to interact with them. They find comfort in holding her hand and reminiscing about happy memories, even though she doesn't respond.

COMPLICATIONS & HEALTH ISSUES

Behavior: Jim, an 88-year-old, experiences frequent infections, weight loss, and other health complications due to his advanced dementia.

Impact: His caregivers work closely with healthcare providers to mange his symptoms and ensure he is comfortable. The focus shifts to palliative care, emphasizing comfort and quality of life.

These examples show how dementia progresses from mild forgetfulness and confusion to severe cognitive and physical decline, highlighting the increasing need for support and care at each stage.

MEDICATION MANAGEMENT

Managing medicines is a critical aspect of caregiving. Older adults often take many medications, which can lead to severe issues if not handled correctly. Be sure to do the following to carefully manage your aging loved ones' medications.

- **Create a Schedule**: Keep track of when and how each medicine should be taken.

- **Use Pill Organizers**: These help prevent missed or doubled doses.

- **Know the Medicines**: Understand what each medicine does, its side effects, and how it interacts with other drugs or foods.

- **Review with Doctors**: Regularly check with healthcare providers to make sure all medicines are still needed, and dosages are correct.

MONITORING HEALTH

Watching for changes in health is key to early problem detection. Keep a close eye on the following key areas of your parents' health.

- **Physical Health**: Regularly check blood pressure, blood sugar levels, and weight. Notice changes in mobility, appetite, and energy.

- **Emotional Health**: Be aware of signs of depression, anxiety, or social withdrawal. Changes in mood and sleep patterns are important to watch.

- **Cognitive Health**: Look for changes in memory and problem-solving. Keep notes on these changes to share with doctors.

EMERGENCY PREPAREDNESS

Being ready for emergencies is crucial. Understand that emergencies can and will happen. Your preparation and readiness for such emergencies can make a difference between life and death. Be sure you have the following in place and at the ready for your loved one.

- **Have a Plan**: Know what to do in case of falls, heart attacks, or strokes. Learn basic first aid and CPR (Cardiopulmonary Resuscitation).

- **Emergency Kit**: Prepare a kit including a list of medicines, medical history, insurance information and contact numbers.

- **Know Your Resources**: Familiarize yourself with the nearest hospital or urgent care center.

CONCLUSION

Understanding your parents' medical and health needs is essential for good caregiving. By learning about common health issues, managing medicines, watching for health changes, and being prepared for emergencies, you can provide better care. This knowledge helps you feel more confident and ensures your parents get the best care possible, improving their quality of life.

CHAPTER 5

FINANCIAL PLANNING AND MANAGEMENT

Taking care of aging parents can be expensive. Planning and managing money well helps make sure you and your parents can handle these costs without too much stress. This chapter covers budgets, understanding insurance and benefits, and finding financial help.

BUDGETING FOR CARE

Making a budget is the first and a very important step. A budget lists all the money that comes in and goes out.

- **Income**: Write down all sources of income, like pensions, social security, savings, and any money from family members.

- **Expenses**: List all expenses, like rent, utilities, insurance, groceries, transportation, and medical costs.

- **Unexpected Costs**: Include extra money for emergencies, like sudden medical bills or home repairs.

Tracking your expenses can help you see where you can save money and make sure you have enough for everything.

INSURANCE & BENEFITS

Understanding insurance and benefits can help cover caregiving costs.

MEDICARE

Medicare is a health insurance program for people aged 65 and older and some younger people with disabilities. This insurance has different "parts" that cover hospital care, medical services, and prescription drugs. Knowing what each part covers can help you plan for medical costs. Here's a simple guide on how to get Medicare:

1. **Check Eligibility**

   You are eligible for Medicare if you are 65 or older, or under 65 with certain disabilities, or have End-Stage Renal Disease (permanent kidney failure requiring dialysis or a transplant).

2. **Understand the Parts of Medicare**

   Medicare Part A: Hospital insurance that helps cover inpatient care, nursing facility care, hospice, and some home health care.

   Medicare Part B: Medical insurance that helps cover doctors' services, outpatient care, medical supplies, and preventive services.

   Medicare Part C (Medicare Advantage): An alternative to Original Medicare that includes Part A, Part B, and sometimes Part D, offered by private companies.

   Medicare Part D: Prescription drug coverage.

3. **Sign Up for Medicare**

   Automatic Enrollment: If you're already receiving Social Security benefits or Railroad Retirement Board benefits, you'll be automatically enrolled in Medicare Parts A and B when you turn 65.

   Manual Enrollment: If you're not automatically enrolled, you'll need to sign up. You can do this during the initial enrollment period, which starts three months before you turn 65 and ends three months after you turn 65.

4. **Ways to Apply**

   Online: Visit the Social Security Administration's website to apply online (www.ssa.gov).

   By Phone: Call the Social Security office at 1-800-772-1213 to apply over the phone.

   In-Person: Visit your local Social Security office to apply in person.

5. **Decide on Additional Coverage**

   Medigap: If you choose Original Medicare (Parts A and B), you might want to buy a Medigap policy from a private company to help pay for costs that Medicare doesn't cover, like copayments, coinsurance, and deductibles.

   Medicare Advantage (Part C): If you prefer, you can choose a Medicare Advantage plan that includes Parts A, B, and sometimes D. These plans are offered by private companies approved by Medicare.

6. **Enroll in Medicare Part D (if needed)**

   If you need prescription drug coverage, you can enroll in a Medicare Part D plan. You can do this during your initial enrollment period or during the annual open enrollment period from October 15 to December 7.

7. **Annual Enrollment**

   Every year, you have the option to make changes to your Medicare plan during the open enrollment period (October 15 to December 7). Review your plan and make any necessary changes.

8. **Receive Your Medicare Card**

   After you sign up, you'll receive a red, white, and blue Medicare card in the mail. This card will show your Medicare number and the parts of Medicare you are enrolled in (Part A, Part B, etc.).

By following these steps, you can sign up for Medicare and ensure you have the coverage you need.

MEDICAID

Medicaid exists for low-income individuals and covers long-term care, which Medicare doesn't fully cover. Applying for Medicaid can help cover healthcare costs for your aging parents. Each state has different rules, so check local regulations. Here's a simple guide on how to apply:

1. **Check Eligibility**

   Medicaid is for people with low income. Check if your parents meet the income and asset limits in your state. Each state has different rules, so you'll need to find the specific requirements for where you live.

2. **Gather Necessary Documents**

   You'll need important documents to apply. Collect documents such as:

   - **Proof of income (pay stubs, Social Security statements)**
   - **Bank Statements**
   - **Proof of Residency (utility bills, lease agreements)**
   - **Identification (birth certificate, driver's license)**
   - **Medical records (if applying for long-term care)**

3. **Complete the Application**

   You can apply for Medicaid in several ways:

   Online: Visit your state's Medicaid website and fill out the application form.

By Phone: Call your state's Medicaid office and apply over the phone.

In-Person: Go to your local Medicaid office or health department to apply in person.

4. **Submit the Application**

    After filling out the application, submit it along with all the required documents. If you apply online or by phone, you might need to mail or upload the documents separately.

5. **Wait for Approval**

    Once you've submitted the application, the Medicaid office will review it. This process can take several weeks. They might contact you if they need more information.

6. **Receive Your Benefits**

    If approved, you'll receive a Medicaid card in the mail. This card can be used to access healthcare services covered by Medicaid.

7. **Follow Up**

    If your application is denied, you can appeal the decision. Contact your state's Medicaid office for information on how to appeal.

8. **Renew Your Coverage**

    Medicaid requires annual renewals to ensure you still meet the eligibility requirements. Make sure to submit renewal forms and documents on time each year.

By following these steps, you can apply for Medicaid to help cover your parents' healthcare needs.

VETERANS' BENEFITS

If your parent served in the military, they might get health care, disability compensation, and pensions. These benefits can be very helpful.

FINANCIAL ASSISTANCE

There are programs that can help with caregiving costs.

- **Government Programs**: These might include direct payments to caregivers, help with home modifications, and medical expense assistance. Check with the Department of Health and Human Services or local aging agencies.

- **Nonprofit Organizations**: Groups like the National Council on Aging (NCOA) provide information on financial help. Disease-specific organizations, like the Alzheimer's Association, offer grants for families.

- **Long-Term Care Insurance**: This can help pay for in-home care, assisted living, and nursing home care. It can be expensive but provides long-term financial help.

LEGAL & ESTATE PLANNING

Planning for the future is important. Consider the following to ensure your parents' legal documents and estate are in order.

- **Legal Documents**: Make sure your parents have wills, powers of attorney, and advance directives. These documents prevent problems later.

- **Elder Law Attorney**: A lawyer can help manage assets, protect against financial abuse, and plan for long-term care.

CONCLUSION

Good financial planning is important for caregiving. By making a budget, understanding insurance, finding financial help, and planning legally, you can handle the financial challenges effectively. This helps you focus on giving the best care to your parents and improves their well-being.

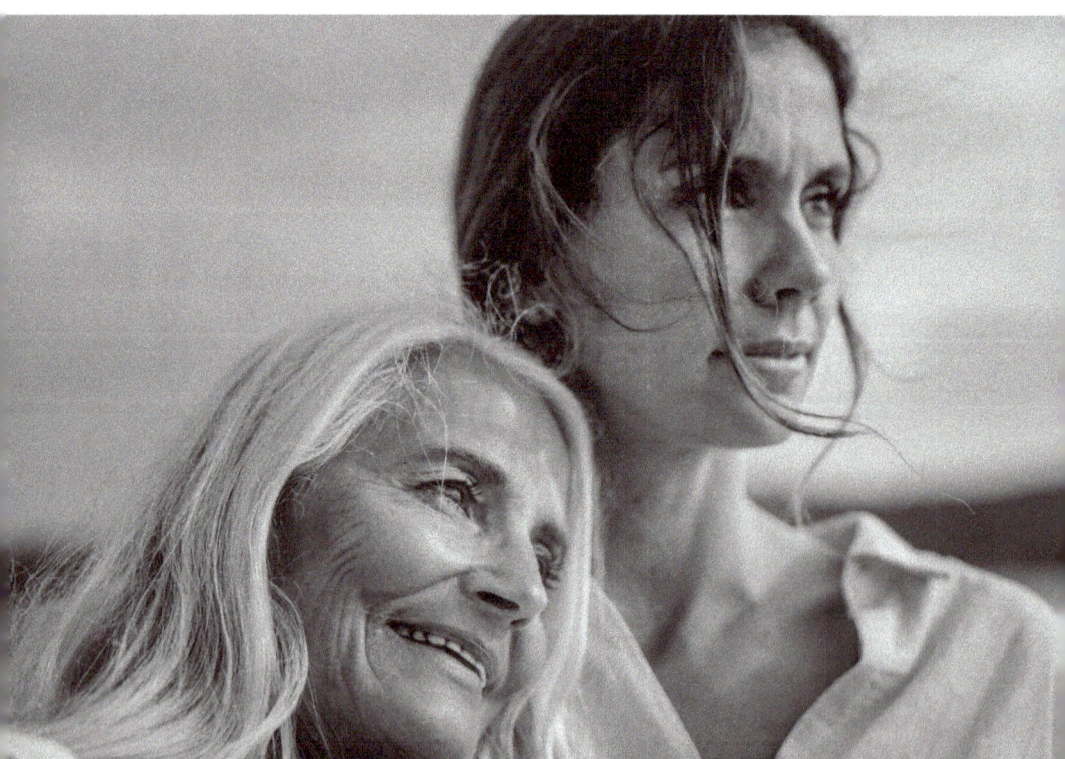

CHAPTER 6

BALANCING WORK, LIFE, AND CAREGIVING

Taking care of your parents while working and managing your own life can be tough. This chapter will help you find ways to manage your time, get support from your boss, and share responsibilities to keep things balanced and avoid getting too stressed out.

TIME MANAGEMENT TECHNIQUES

Managing your time well is very important when you have to take care of your parents, manage work, and all the responsibility of your own life. Here are some tips.

- **Prioritize Tasks**: Do the most important things first each day, like going to the doctor, giving medicine, or finishing work projects.

- **Create a Routine**: Having a daily routine helps both you and your parents feel more organized and less worried.

- **Set Realistic Goals**: Don't try to do too much. It's okay if not everything is perfect. Just do your best.

- **Use Tools and Apps**: Use calendars and reminder apps to keep track of appointments and tasks. Share them with family members to stay coordinated.

The following are just some of the many calendar and reminder apps that can help you keep track of your parents' appointments and tasks:

CALENDAR APPS

App: Google Calendar
Features: Syncs with other Google services, shareable with family members, set reminders, color-code events.
Platforms: iOS, Android, Web

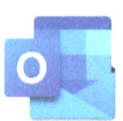

App: Apple (iOS) Calendar
Features: Integrated with iOS devices, Siri integration, shareable with family, set alerts.
Platforms: iOS, macOS

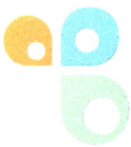

App: Microsoft Outlook > Calendar
Features: Integrated with email, set reminders, share calendars, color-code events.
Platforms: iOS, Android, Web, Windows

App: Cozi Family Organizer
Features: Shared family calendar, to-do lists, shopping lists, reminders.
Platforms: iOS, Android, Web

REMINDER APPS

App: ToDoist
Features: Task lists, set reminders, share tasks, organize by projects, sync across devices.
Platforms: iOS, Android, Web, macOS, Windows

App: Microsoft To Do
Features: Task lists, reminders, integrate with Microsoft services (calendar, email, etc.), share tasks.
Platforms: iOS, Android, Web, macOS, Windows

App: Any.Do
Features: Task lists, calendar integration, reminders, share tasks, voice entry.
Platforms: iOS, Android, Web, macOS, Windows

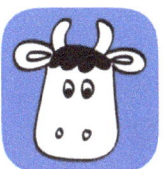

App: Remember the Milk
Features: Task lists, set reminders, organize by tags, sync across devices, share tasks.
Platforms: iOS, Android, Web

COMBINATION APPS (CALENDAR + REMINDER)

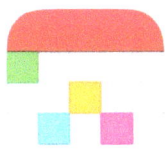

App: Fantastical
Features: Calendar and reminders in one app, natural language input, syncs with multiple calendar services, set alerts.
Platforms: iOS, macOS

App: TimeTree
Features: Shared calendar, reminders, notes, color-code events, sync across devices.
Platforms: iOS, Android, Web

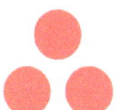

App: Asana
Features: Task and project management, calendar view, set reminders, share tasks, track progress.
Platforms: iOS, Android, Web

Using these apps can help you stay organized and ensure that you don't miss any important appointments or tasks while caring for your parents.

EMPLOYER SUPPORT

Talking to your boss about your caregiving responsibilities can open up the opportunity to better balancing work and caregiving. Here's how:

- **Communicate Needs**: Tell your boss or HR (Human Resources) about your caregiving duties. Being honest can help them understand and support you.

- **Flexible Work Arrangements**: Some jobs offer flexible hours or let you work from home. These options can make it easier to manage caregiving tasks.

- **Family Leave Policies**: Know your company's leave policies. In the U.S., the Family and Medical Leave Act (FMLA) lets eligible workers take unpaid leave to care for family.

- **Employee Assistance Programs (EAPs)**: Some companies have programs that offer counseling and resources for caregivers. These can be very helpful.

DELEGATING RESPONSIBILITIES

Many times, caregiving can be too much for one person. Share the work with others to make it easier.

- **Involve Family Members**: Ask siblings and other relatives to help. Give everyone specific tasks based on what they can do best.

- **Professional Caregivers**: Hiring caregivers can give you a break and make sure your parents get the best care.

- **Community Resources**: Use local services like adult day care centers, meal programs, and transportation services to get extra help.

SELF-CARE AND SETTING BOUNDARIES

To stay healthy and happy, you need to take care of yourself and set limits on what you can do:

- **Self-Care Practices**: Make time for things you enjoy, like exercise, hobbies, and relaxing activities. This helps you stay physically and emotionally healthy.

- **Set Boundaries**: Tell your family what you can and can't do. Make sure you have time for yourself.

- **Seek Support Groups**: Join groups where caregivers share their experiences and advice. It helps to know you're not alone.

CONCLUSION

Balancing work, life, and caregiving takes careful planning and good communication. By managing your time well, getting support from your boss, sharing tasks, and taking care of yourself, you can keep things balanced. This way, you can take good care of your parents while also taking care of yourself.

CHAPTER 7

LEGAL CONSIDERATIONS AND PLANNING

When we take care of our aging parents, we want to make sure they are happy and safe. Sometimes, this means we need to think about important papers and plans that help look after them now and in the future. This chapter will help explain how we can do that in simple ways.

IMPORTANT PAPERS EVERYONE NEEDS

Think of these legal documents as a map that informs how to care for your parents and their belongings in the way they wish prior to their passing:

- **Power of Attorney (POA)**: This is a legal document that lets someone your parents trust to make decisions for them if they ever can't decide for themselves.

- **Living Will**: This document tells doctors what kind of medical help your parents want if they get sick and can't speak for themselves. This often covers your parents' wishes regarding life support and when to end it, when and if the situation calls for it.

- **Will**: This legal document is the formal plan for how your parents' belongings and assets will be handled and passed on when they are no longer here, ensuring they go where the parents wish them to while they are still able to make those decisions.

- **Trusts**: These are legal entities that are reserved for holding your parents' key assets like their house, money and savings, and valuables. A trust helps manage financial assets when they aren't able to do it themselves.

WHEN SOMEONE HAS TO HELP MAKE DECISIONS

Sometimes, if an individual is advanced in age and can't make decisions about their health or money, someone may be granted authority over and responsibility for those decisions:

- **Guardianship**: This is when a court grants an adult with authority and responsibility over their aging parents so that they can make decisions for them because they are no longer competent to make independent decisions themselves.

- **Conservatorship**: Like guardianship, a conservatorship is focused solely on authority over and responsibility for an aging parent's money or property.

PLANNING FOR LATER

Planning is an important step that cannot be overemphasized. It is essential to plan well and as far in advance as possible so that all key pieces of information, legal documents and your parents' wishes are noted.

- **Discuss Wishes and Wants**: It's best to discuss how your parents want things done, from early care as it becomes needed, to end-of-life concerns such as their will, living will, power of attorney, and others. An open and candid conversation does not have to be uncomfortable and is vital to ensuring everyone understands and agrees.

- **Keep Things Updated**: Life changes, like moving into a new house, getting a pet, or births of new family members are important milestones that often mean we need to update the important documents that account for your parents' wishes and how they will be carried out.

- **Getting Help from Experts**: Navigating when and what to create, document and update as your parents age can be both overwhelming and confusing. Reach out and seek help from individuals who know about the rules and documents that need to be in place, like doctors, lawyers, and certified senior advisors (CSA).

BEING KIND AND RESPECTFUL

While sorting out your parents' wishes, wants, and directives regarding their care, belongings, and end-of-life choices, it's important to actively and empathetically listen to your parents and treat them with understanding and kindness. Though these conversations do not have to be difficult, they can sometimes be stressful for both you and your parents. Approach the conversations with empathy so that your parents feel loved and respected throughout the conversation, knowing that their wishes are important to you.

CONCLUSION

Taking care of the legalities and end-of-life choices might sound and feel intrusive, but it is necessary work in order to make sure your parents are cared for and happy. By understanding and organizing these important documents, and having these conversations, you are helping ensure that everything that matters to your parents is in good hands and you are able to see them through.

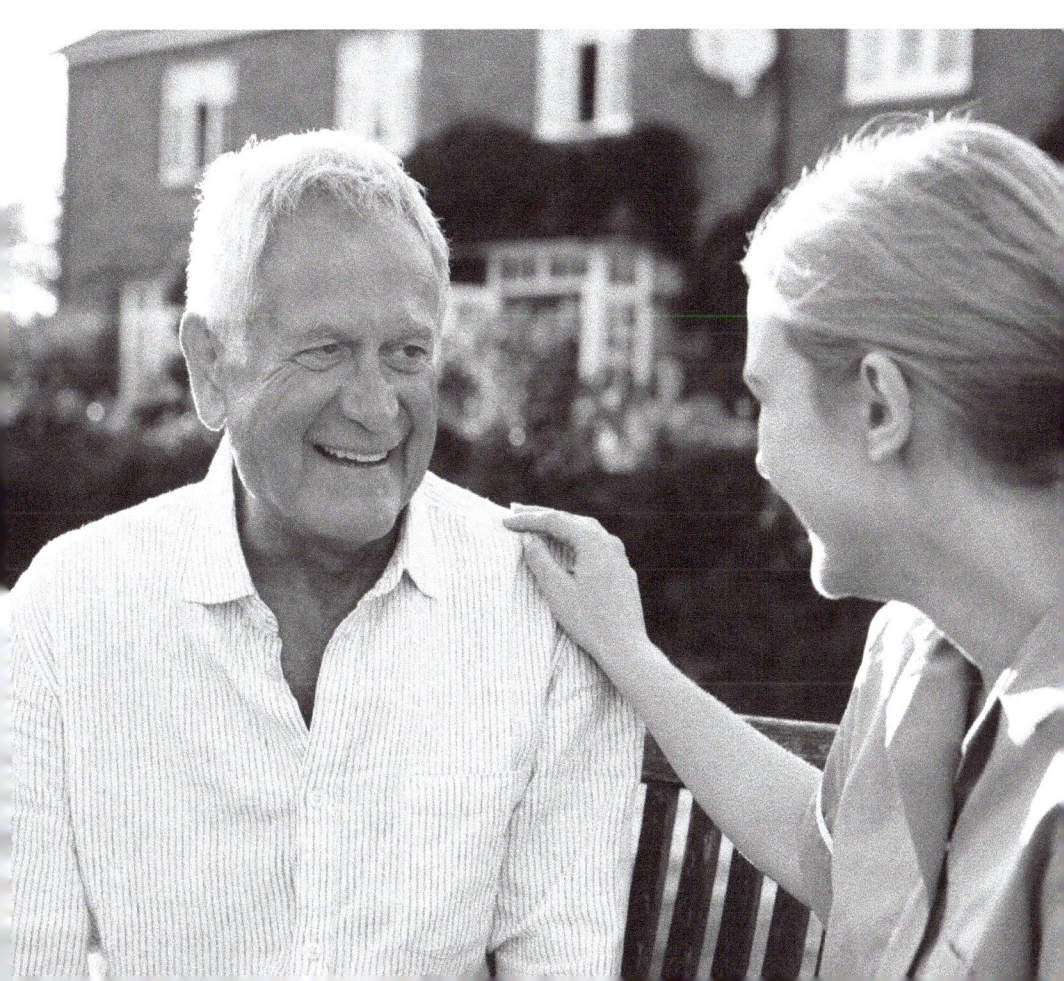

CHAPTER 8

ENHANCING QUALITY OF LIFE

As our parents grow older, we want to make sure they are happy and comfortable. This chapter focuses on how to make your parents' home safer, and ways to help them stay independent for as long as possible.

FALLS

> **Falls are the leading cause of injury and injury-related deaths for adults aged 65 and older.**

Falls are not only the most common cause of injury, they also carry considerable potential costs - both monetarily and in terms of changes to an aging parent's mobility and daily life.

HOW MUCH DO FALLS COST?

Medical Bills:

- In the United States, if an older person falls and gets hurt, it might cost more than $30,000 to help them get better. This includes money for doctors, hospitals, and things they might need at home to move around more easily.

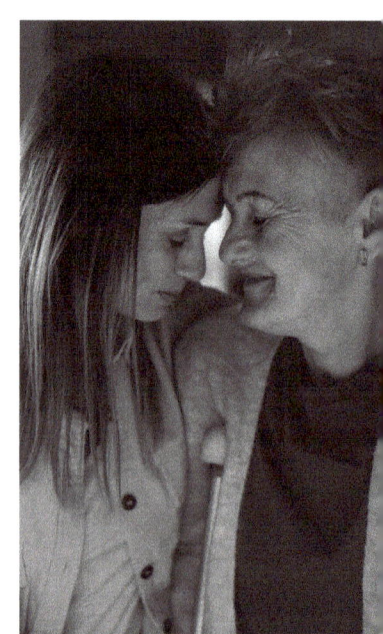

- In other countries, the cost might be different, but it's usually a considerable sum for medical care after a fall.

Other Costs:

- Sometimes family members have to work less to take care of their older loved ones who suffered a fall. This means they might earn less income as a result.
- Families might also spend money in order to make parents' homes safer. This could include adding grab bars in the bathroom, improved lighting to see better, and improvements to entranceways and steps to minimize the chances of future falls.

HOW DO FALLS CHANGE LIVES?

Difficulty in Movement:

- If someone breaks a bone like a hip when they fall, they can expect to not be able to walk or move like they used to. Sometimes, they need many months to recuperate, and they often need help even after they heal.
- Head injuries from falls can be particularly devastating and may cause neurological trauma that can make it difficult for them to think clearly or remember things.

Fear of Falling Again:

- After falling once, some older people might be scared of falling again. This fear can make them less active, which can actually make it *easier* for them to fall again.

Needing More Help:

- After a fall, an older person might need more help from others to do everyday things. This can lead to feelings of sadness or anxiety because they are not as independent as they were before the fall.
- The limited mobility and independence can also lead to feelings

of loneliness and a sense of being "left out" because of the limitations inhibiting what they previously were able to do with family or friends.

STOPPING FALLS BEFORE THEY HAPPEN

Because falls can be so serious, it's important to try to stop them before they happen. The following are some preventative measures that can be taken before a fall ever occurs.

- **Exercise**: Doing exercises that make legs stronger and improve balance can help prevent falls.
- **Making Homes Safer**: Adding things like more lights, grab bars, and non-slip mats can make a home safer for your aging parents.
- **Regular Check-ups**: Going to the doctor to check eyes and vision, and making sure medicines are appropriate and at the right dosages can go a long way to preventing falls.

Falls can be very costly and can change how older people live their lives. By understanding these costs and impacts, and by working to prevent falls, we can help our aging parents stay healthy and happy for as long as possible.

MAKING THE HOME SAFE

Parents might need a little help getting around their house safely as they age. Some tips to safeguard your loved ones by making their home safer include:

- **Remove Trip Hazards**: Make sure there are no loose rugs or wires they can trip over. Keep floors clear and safe.
- **Improve Bathroom Safety**: Install grab bars in the bathroom so

that your parents can move around easily and securely without slipping.

- **Bring Things into Reach**: Make sure things that are used a lot are easy to reach without climbing or bending down excessively.
- **Increase Visibility with Lighting**: Good lighting helps your aging parent see better, especially at night when a significant proportion of falls occur. Install additional night lights in hallways and near stairs.

Creating a safe and comfortable environment for aging parents is a crucial aspect of caregiving. It involves making necessary home modifications, ensuring safety, and fostering an atmosphere of comfort and dignity. The remainder of this chapter explores practical steps to adapt the living space, enhance safety measures, and promote a sense of well-being and security for aging parents.

COMMON HOME MODIFICATIONS

As parents age, their physical capabilities often change, necessitating adjustments to the living environment to ensure safety and accessibility. The following are some of the most common home modifications:

- **Fall Prevention**: As we've already seen, falls are a significant risk for older adults. Install grab bars in bathrooms near toilets and showers, add non-slip mats, and ensure that all rugs are secured to the floor. Staircases should have sturdy handrails, and well-lit paths should be maintained throughout the house.
- **Mobility Enhancements**: For parents with mobility issues, consider installing ramps for wheelchair access and stairlifts for multi-level homes. Widening doorways can accommodate walkers and wheelchairs.

- **Bathroom Safety**: Bathrooms are often the most hazardous areas in the home. Installing a walk-in shower, adding a shower seat, and ensuring easy access to toiletries can make daily routines safer. Elevated toilet seats and grab bars can also provide additional support.

- **Lighting**: Good lighting is essential for preventing accidents. Ensure all areas of the home are well-lit, particularly hallways, staircases, and outdoor spaces. Nightlights can help older adults navigate their home at night.

HOME SAFETY CHECKLIST FOR THE ELDERLY AND DISABLED

GENERAL HOME SAFETY

- **Clear Pathways**:
  - [ ] Ensure all walkways inside and outside the home are clear of obstacles and clutter.

- **Adequate Lighting**:
  - [ ] Install bright lights in all rooms, hallways, and entryways. Consider night lights in bedrooms and bathrooms.

- **Secure Rugs**:
  - [ ] Use non-slip pads under all rugs or remove loose rugs altogether to prevent tripping and falls.

- **Emergency Numbers**:
  - [ ] Keep a list of emergency contact numbers in large print by each phone or in a central location.

BATHROOM SAFETY

- **Grab Bars:**
  - [ ] Install grab bars in the shower, bathtub, and near the toilet to help prevent falls.
- **Non-Slip Mats**:
  - [ ] Place non-slip mats in the bathtub and on shower floors.
- **Raised Toilet Seat**:
  - [ ] Use a raised toilet seat with armrests to assist those with mobility issues.
- **Shower Seat**:
  - [ ] Provide a stable shower seat to enable bathing without standing.

KITCHEN SAFETY

- **Accessible Storage:**
  - [ ] Keep frequently used items in easy-to-reach locations, avoiding the need to use step stools or ladders.
- **Automatic Shut-off Appliances**:
  - [ ] Use appliances that automatically shut off, such as kettles and irons, to prevent accidents such as burns and fires.
- **Non-Slip Flooring**:
  - [ ] Ensure kitchen floors are non-slip or use non-slip mats where spills are likely.
- **Clear Cooking Areas**:
  - [ ] Keep cooking areas clear of flammable materials like towels and paper.

BEDROOM SAFETY

- **Accessible Bed Height:**
  - ☐ Ensure the bed is at a height that is easy to get in and out of.

- **Bed Rails**:
  - ☐ Consider installing bed rails to provide support for getting in and out of bed.

- **Night Light**:
  - ☐ Place a night light in the bedroom to make it easier to see at night.

- **Cordless Phone**:
  - ☐ Keep a cordless phone or mobile phone near the bed for easy access to communication.

LIVING AREA SAFETY

- **Sturdy Furniture**:
  - ☐ Use sturdy furniture that is easy to get in and out of and won't tip over easily.

- **Cord Management**:
  - ☐ Secure cords to the wall or hide them under furniture to prevent tripping.

- **Good Seating Support**:
  - ☐ Chairs and sofas should have good back support and not be too low to the ground.

- **Remote Controls**:
  - ☐ Keep remote controls for the television and other devices within easy reach.

STAIRWAY AND HALLWAY SAFETY

- **Handrails**:
  - [ ] Install handrails on both sides of stairways.
- **Good Lighting**:
  - [ ] Ensure stairways and hallways are well-lit.
- **Step Visibility**:
  - [ ] Mark the edges of steps with contrasting tape to make them more visible.
- **Clutter-Free**:
  - [ ] Keep stairs and hallways clear of any items to avoid tripping hazards.

OUTDOOR SAFETY

- **Secure Railings**:
  - [ ] Check that all outdoor railings are secure and sturdy.
- **Smooth Pathways**:
  - [ ] Repair any uneven surfaces or cracks in pathways.
- **Adequate Lighting**:
  - [ ] Ensure that all outdoor areas are well-lit, especially the entrances.
- **Non-slip Surfaces**:
  - [ ] Apply non-slip paint or strips to steps or porches.

Using this checklist regularly can help maintain a safe and comfortable home environment for the elderly and disabled, promoting their independence and well-being.

SAFETY MEASURES

Beyond physical modifications, implementing comprehensive safety measures is vital for creating a secure living environment:

- **Emergency Preparedness**: Have a plan in place for emergencies. Ensure that smoke detectors and carbon monoxide alarms are installed and functioning correctly. Keep emergency numbers easily accessible, and consider using medical alert systems that allow aging parents to call for help if needed.

- **Medication Management**: Properly organizing and storing medications can prevent accidental overdoses or missed doses. Use pill organizers, set up reminders, and keep a list of all medications, dosages, and schedules in an easily accessible place.

- **Fire Safety**: Ensure that the home has working fire extinguishers, and teach everyone how to use them. Develop and practice an emergency exit plan with your aging parents.

- **Security**: Secure the home against potential intruders. Install locks on windows and doors, consider a home security system, and ensure that your parents know how to use it.

CREATING COMFORT

Beyond safety, creating a comfortable and welcoming environment is essential for the emotional and mental well-being of aging parents:

- **Personalization**: Personalize their living space with familiar items, such as photos, favorite books, and cherished mementos. These items can provide comfort and a sense of continuity.

- **Comfortable Furniture**: Ensure that furniture is comfortable and accessible. Recliners, lift chairs, and beds with adjustable features can make daily living more comfortable and support physical needs.

- **Temperature Control**: Aging parents may be more sensitive to cold. Be sure the temperature of the home is adjusted to a comfortable temperature for them.

CONCLUSION

Making life great for aging parents means helping them stay active and safe. By creating a safe environment that allows for your parents' independence, actively making their home safer, and safeguarding against falls, you can help them live a more secure and safe existence.

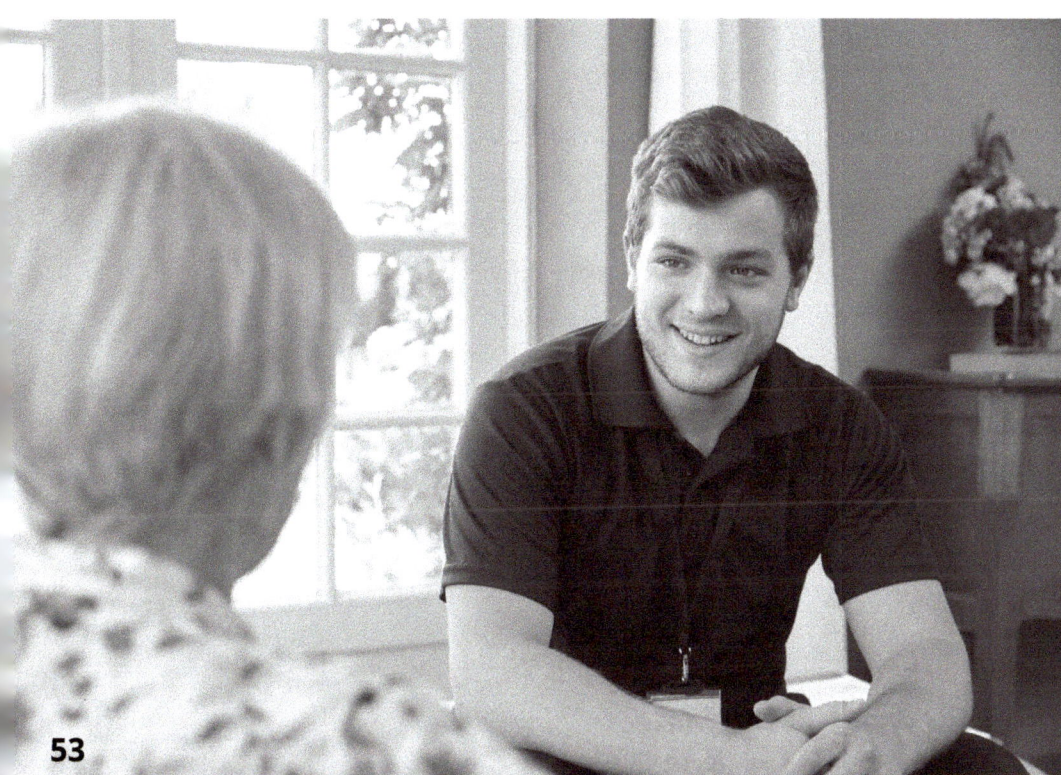

CHAPTER 9
KEEPING IN TOUCH AND STAYING HAPPY

Depression is not a normal part of aging! Taking care of your parents means helping them stay connected with friends and family and keeping their minds happy and healthy. This chapter discusses why it's important for your aging parents to have friends and fun activities, and what we can do if they feel sad or worried.

WHEN AGING PARENTS FEEL SAD OR WORRIED

Sometimes, aging parents might feel sad or anxious. It's important to know the signs and help them reconcile their emotions to feel better:

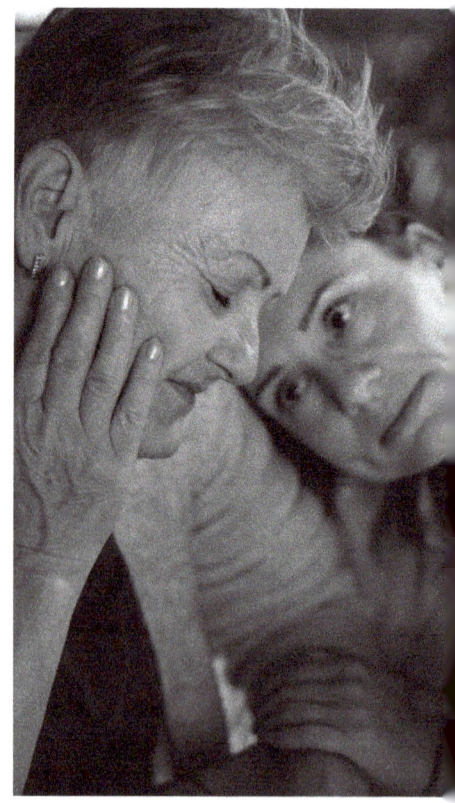

- **Sadness:** If your parents seem depressed, aren't enjoying the things they usually enjoy, or appear to be tired much or all of the time, they might be experiencing feelings of sadness.
- **Anxiety**: If your parents seem overly worried, can't relax, or are experiencing restlessness to the extent that it interferes with their happiness and well-being, they might be experiencing anxiety.

- **Forgetfulness**: If you parents are noticeably and increasingly forgetting things, getting confused, or having trouble with everyday tasks, it's important to notice and help them.

HELPING THEM FEEL BETTER

The following are ways you can help your parents stay mentally healthy and happy.

- **Daily Routine**: Having a regular schedule can make parents feel safe and organized. Make sure they have fun activities and plenty of rest every day.
- **Staying Active**: Encourage your parents to move around and stay active. Light movement such as going for a walk, an easy swim, or doing light yoga are good options for keeping your parents active. This is not only good for their bodies but also helps their mood.
- **Getting Help**: If you notice your parents are often sad, worried, or confused, it might be time to talk to someone who can help, like a doctor or counselor.
- **Having Support**: Check in with your parents often, listen to their stories and worries, and let them know you are there to help and care for them. Their knowledge and confidence in you for support can do wonders for their mental state.
- **Relaxing**: Teach your parents simple ways to relax, like breathing exercises or listening to calm music or sounds. This can alleviate stress and improve their mental state.

MAKING HOME A HAPPY PLACE

Making sure your parents' home is a happy place is extremely important to health and well-being. This means not only enhancing the space to be personalized and uplifting, but also that it should be a place of frequent positive talks, sharing of good news, and a place where you do fun things together. Maintain empathy and always speak kindly during conversations or chats. And maintain positive involvement by making sure your parents feel involved in family decisions.

WHY FRIENDS ARE IMPORTANT

Having friends and doing fun things together with them is a boost for everyone, especially your aging parents. It makes them feel loved and important, which, in turn, improves their happiness. When they join clubs, go to community events, or hang out at senior centers, they meet new people and have fun too.

FUN ACTIVITIES FOR OLDER ADULTS

There are lots of ways to help your parents stay active and enjoy their time:

- **Joining in the Community**: Encourage them to go to events or places where they can meet other people. This could be a game night at the community center or a gardening club.
- **Enjoying Hobbies**: Plan time to do things they love, like painting, gardening, or playing cards. Doing things they enjoy can make them very happy.
- **Using Technology**: Teach your parents how to use a smartphone, tablet, or computer. This way, they can chat with family and friends who live far away, watch their favorite shows, or even join groups online.
- **Moving Around**: Encourage them to walk or do simple stretches. This keeps their muscles strong and helps them stay balanced.
- **Brain Games**: Puzzles, reading books, or even learning something new on a computer can keep their minds sharp and active.

- **Helping Others**: Sometimes, parents enjoy helping out in the community, like at food banks or libraries, which makes them feel happy and useful.
- **Family Time**: Having family over for dinner or visiting them on weekends can help your parents feel connected. If you can, visit your parents often or call them if they live far away. Just hearing your voice can make them very happy.

CONCLUSION

Keeping in touch with others and supporting mental health are very important for taking care of parents. By helping them stay connected, noticing when they feel sad or worried, and doing fun activities, you can make their life happier and more fulfilling. This not only makes them feel better but also strengthens your relationship with them, making every day more enjoyable for everyone.

CHAPTER 10

PLANNING FOR THE FUTURE

When we take care of older parents, we also have to think about how to make their later years as happy and comfortable as possible. This chapter discusses planning ahead for advanced age, declining health, and how to care for your parents at the end of their life.

PLANNING AHEAD

Talking and planning ahead helps make sure that we can care for our parents the way they would want:

- **Making Plans:** It's like writing down a list of instructions for what your parents would want if they become too sick to tell the doctor themselves. This includes which medicines they want or don't want.

- **Talking About Their Wishes**: It's really important to talk to your parents about what they want when they are very old or sick. Ask them about things like whether they want to stay at home if they get very ill and how they feel about hospitals.

- **Keeping Plans Updated**: Sometimes what your parents want might change, especially if they get sick. Make sure to talk about their wishes often and update any plans to match what they now want.

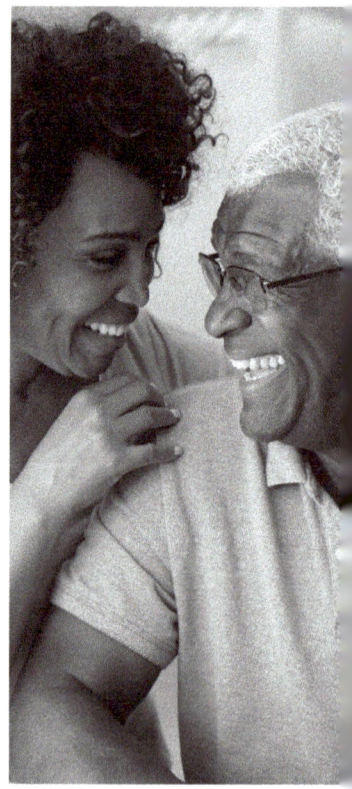

SUPPORTING EACH OTHER

The end of someone's life can be a sad and difficult time, but there are ways to make it a little easier:

- **Talking and Sharing**: Let your parents talk about how they feel and what they're scared of. Listen to them and let them know it's okay to share their feelings.

- **Making Memories Last**: Help your parents leave behind memories like writing letters, making scrapbooks, or recording stories about their life. This way, you can remember them and keep their stories alive.

- **Getting Help for Yourself**: Taking care of someone at the end of their life is hard. It's okay for caregivers to need a break and talk to friends, family, or counselors about how they're feeling.

PROFESSIONAL CAREGIVERS AND NURSING HOMES

Taking care of older parents can be an enormous job, and sometimes you might need help from professionals or even think about a place like a nursing home for them to live. It's important to know when it's time to get this help and how to do it. This will make sure your parents are happy and healthy and that you can manage everything they need without becoming overwhelmed.

WHEN TO HIRE PROFESSIONAL CAREGIVERS

- **Too Much to Handle Alone**: If you start feeling really overwhelmed with taking care of your parents, and it's too much to do by yourself, it might be time to get some help.

- **Medical Needs**: Sometimes, older people need special medical care that you might not know how to give. Professional caregivers know how to take care of these needs safely.

- **You Need a Break**: Taking care of someone all the time can exhaust a person. Hiring a caregiver can give you time to rest and do other important things, so you can come back feeling refreshed.

- **Safety Concerns**: If it's hard for your parents to move around without falling or getting hurt, a professional caregiver can help make sure they are safe.

HOW TO HIRE PROFESSIONAL CAREGIVERS

- **Find the Right People**: You can look for caregivers by talking to friends who have hired someone before, or by looking online at trusted websites. There are companies that find caregivers for you and make sure they are good at their job and are kind to your parents.

- **Interview Them**: Just as when someone pursues any job, you should interview caregivers to gauge if they are friendly and if they know how to take care of your parents' specific needs.

- **Check Their Background**: It's very important to make sure that the person who will be looking after your parents is trustworthy and has the right skills. The companies that help find caregivers can check this for you.

- **Try It Out**: Sometimes, you can have a caregiver start by working just a few hours to see how they get along with your parents. If your parents like them and you think they do a good job, you can increase the hours they work.

WHEN IT MIGHT BE TIME FOR A NURSING HOME

- **Medical Care**: If your parents need a lot of medical care spanning day and night, a nursing home might be the best place for them. Nursing homes have doctors and nurses staffed around the clock.
- **Safety**: If it's very hard for your parents to do everyday things like walking, eating, or taking a bath, even with help at home, a nursing home can make sure they are safe and well-cared for.
- **Too Hard at Home**: Sometimes, even with a caregiver, it can be too difficult to take care of your parents at home because they need special equipment or lots of help that you can't provide there.

HOW TO CHOOSE A NURSING HOME

- **Visit Different Places**: Look at different nursing homes with your family. See which ones are clean, friendly, and have good activities that your parents might enjoy.
- **Talk to Staff and Residents**: Ask the people who work there and the people who live there what they think about the place. This can help you decide if it's a happy and healthy place for your parents.
- **Think About What Your Parents Like**: Consider what kinds of things your parents like to do and if the nursing home has activities they would enjoy. It's important that they feel happy and have fun activities to participate in.

DIFFERENT TYPES OF CARE

There are special ways to care for people when they are very sick and not going to get better.

- **Palliative Care**: This is a special kind of care that helps make sick people feel better by taking away pain and discomfort. It's not just for people who are at the end of their life; it can be for anyone who is very sick.

- **Hospice Care**: This type of care is given when doctors say that a person might only have six months or less to live. It helps them feel comfortable and takes care of them mostly at home, not in a hospital. The focus is on making sure they are as happy and pain-free as possible.

When should you think about palliative or hospice care? If your parents are getting very sick, it might be time to talk about these types of care. Doctors and nurses can help decide when it's time to start thinking about palliative care or hospice.

CONCLUSION

Whether getting a caregiver to help at home or thinking about a nursing home, making sure your parents are taken care of is very important. Remember, asking for help is okay and can make things better for both you and your parents. It means that your parents will get the care they need, and you still have time to take care of yourself. Planning for the future and taking care of parents at the end of their life are important tasks. By talking about plans early, understanding different types of care, and supporting each other, you can help make your parents' final years full of dignity and comfort. This careful planning and kind of care can make the last part of their lives special and peaceful.

FINAL THOUGHTS

The information in this guide serves as a foundational starting point, offering the essential first steps for addressing your parents' unique circumstances. However, every family situation is different, and navigating the complexities of aging requires a tailored approach. For a more comprehensive and personalized plan that addresses the specific needs of your aging parents, it is highly recommended that you consult a qualified professional, such as a Certified Senior Advisor (CSA). These experts can help you develop a detailed, customized strategy that considers all aspects of your parents' well-being, from healthcare and finances to daily living arrangements and long-term planning.

ABOUT CARING HANDS

Founded by Registered Nurses who wanted to make a difference in the community in which they lived and served, Caring Hands Home Health, Inc. is an award-winning and leading Home Care service provider serving the Triad, Triangle, Charlotte, and other areas of North Carolina. Since 2002, Caring Hands Home Health has provided North Carolina with superior care to the elderly and disabled members of the community, easing the process of finding the best care providers and offering incomparable solutions that empower the elderly and disabled to feel more independent, safe, and happy through high quality Home Care service within the comfort of their homes. Learn more about Caring Hands at www.caringhandshhc.com.

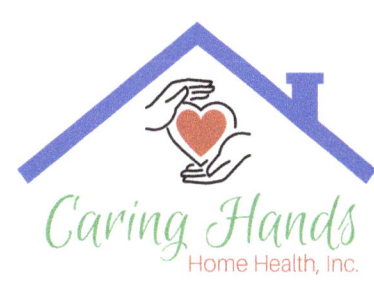

ABOUT THE AUTHOR

Richele Wilkins, RN, BSN, is a senior care advisor and 28+ year veteran of the caregiving industry. A frequent international public speaker for caregivers and the caregiving industry, Richele has spent close to 30 years in the business of intimately knowing the needs of seniors and creating safe and happy accommodations and caregiving situations for them. As a much sought-after expert, coach, and leader of the caregiving industry, she has made it her mission to help caregivers around the globe better prepare for and provide care to aging and disabled loved ones across a range of care environments from home care to palliative care and beyond.

Richele spends her days working within her own award-winning caregiving company, Caring Hands Home Health, Inc., on the road speaking at caregiver and leadership conferences, or spending time with her son and mother.

You can arrange an appointment to speak with Richele or her staff at her company's website, caringhandshhc.com.

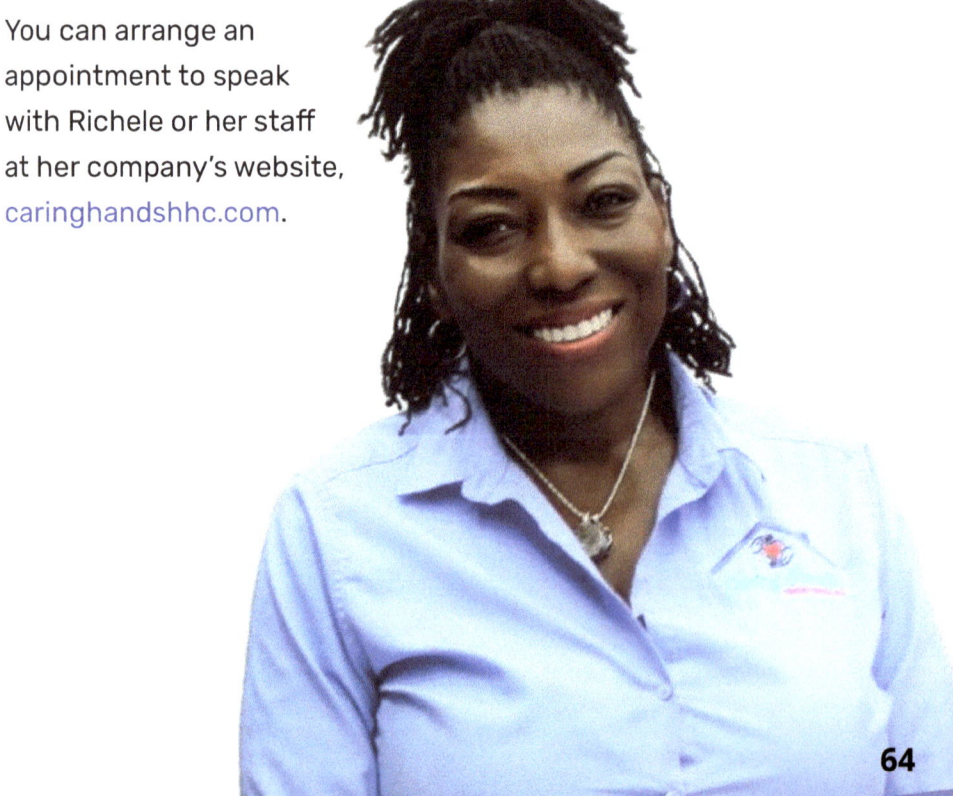

www.ingramcontent.com/pod-product-compliance
Lightning Source LLC
Chambersburg PA
CBHW052033030426
42337CB00027B/4994